The HEALTHY WHOLE *RX*

The HEALTHY WHOLE *RX*

Connecting Physical, Spiritual &
Cognitive Health to Achieve Wholeness
and Maintain Wellbeing

SABINE D. ELISEE, DO, MPH

purposely created
PUBLISHING

THE HEALTHY WHOLE RX

Published by Purposely Created Publishing Group™

Printed in the United States of America

ISBN: 978-1-64484-203-4

The Healthy Whole Rx is dedicated to my family, who brings wholeness to my life. My husband Vicly; my three boys Bay, Blakie, and Brax; my mom and dad Reverend & Mrs. Delinois; and my siblings Nathan, Tania, Pierry, and Stefie—each of you are the wind in my sail that collectively set me in motion. I love you. To my grandmother Meme, whose memory will never fade. Meme, you were the tangible presence of love while living out your journey of life on this earth. May I continue your legacy and be the tangible presence of Love.

Table of Contents

Foreword

Being the eldest brother of the author, I could always plainly see her passion for helping others. Dr. Elisee has always played the role of listening ear, support system, advisor, and when necessary, advocate. These are the same qualities that have taken her on to journeys within the medical fields with that same goal to be that outstretched arm always willing to help her fellow human being.

Her goal is to focus on total health and to help in the healing and maintaining of positive states of being for the entire human condition. This same approach led her to study Osteopathic Medicine. It also keeps her on the forefront of new trends, data, and discoveries in medicine.

Within these pages, Dr. Elisee will address topics such as mental health, physical health, spiritual health, and stress that together will paint a picture of health for the "whole person."

Nathan Delinois
(artist Nate Dee)

Introduction

The purpose of the *Healthy Whole Rx* is to keep people from living fragmented, disconnected lifestyles that hinder their overall wellbeing and daily productivity. As a doctor, I speak to people from various backgrounds and walks in life. I count it a privilege in having the opportunity to peek into the often-hidden frailty of man. Throughout the years of patient encounters and speaking at small group forums or congregation-sized assemblies, a recurrent premise would emerge—brokenness. People are broken, fragmented, holding onto and addressing only part of the solution. I meet people in health clubs who regularly address their physical health but overlook their spiritual health and cognitive health. In religious or spiritual settings, wholeheartedly there is a genuine pursuit to strengthen spiritual health but oftentimes, little to no attention is placed on the necessity to engage physical health or cognitive health. And as you can imagine, there are times when I walk the warm beaches of South Florida and meet individuals who have just completed their peaceful morning hour of mindful meditation with the grains of sand under their feet in the perfect place to perceive the beauty of nature. As my conversations with some of these new friends continue, it is apparent that while much attention is given to the cultivation of cognitive health, the necessity to feed physical health and spiritual health is discounted. Each one of these assemblies have maximized and insulated that one specific area of health. While in and of itself this is great, it is not enough. The need for wholeness in our health makes sense. Wholeness in our health is available to everyone. But it is only attainable when you actively and regularly engage to integrate the three components of health. This book teaches practical steps that reconnect the three components of your health—physical, spiritual, and cognitive. Learn the Healthy Whole Rx and bring wholeness to your health.

CHAPTER I

The Achilles Heel of Strength

The name Sabine means strength and beauty. I love my name—well, at least now I do. Growing up, I had plans to change my name because I was called "Soybean," "Soggy Bean," "String Bean," and any other bean that you can think of. Little did I know that the meaning of my name, strength, would permeate my personality and nature. As human beings, we are designed in a fashion that when mishap, misfortune, or tragedy occurs, we mount up a response that often we did not realize was wrapped deep in the chambers of our core. For the indecisive person, it is only in a moment of panic that they have the wherewithal to make a quick decision that ultimately is the right decision. As for me, when faced with a difficult situation, my default nature of strength triggers me to push through with tenacity and determination.

But at what cost? While strength is a virtuous attribute, it can present with a detrimental self-sacrificing resolve to succeed and "push through" no matter what.

As I now realize, this is what occurred in my life during my high school years when my grandmother was diagnosed with pancreatic cancer. Strength was on display, but a despondent Sabine was functioning. Years later, a similar event occurred, an image of strength but agony within when faced with the unexpected in my first year of medical school. In Haiti, there is a common adage that states, "Life says, 'Let's go,' but it will never tell you where you are going or what path it will take." As one who continuously studies the body, I have learned that there remains a constant necessity. Any distress that occurs in life—physical or emotional—must be identified and appropriately addressed. If not, it will continue to reproduce itself as a different toxic fruit all from the same root. When we are hit with the calamities of life yet maintain the ability to operate and maintain peak performance, we call it strength. And to some extent, maybe it is, but truly, the mission behind that perceived "strength" is avoidance—actively not addressing the sadness and disappointment of what naturally occurs in life, like sickness or death. Seeing my grandmother's round, plump, pecan-brown cheeks thin out, her voice progressively become weak, and her hand grow frail set forth gusts of distressing, agitating, torrential winds in the heart and mind of a sixteen-year-old who was hit with life. I internalized that distress. I choose to shift my focus in hopes of ignoring a covert but growing despair that was within. To further engage in studies, work, or anything else that could keep my mind distracted and my energy focused away from the reality I faced when entering the doors of 7611—my childhood home. And even as adults, many of us continue to disengage and fix our focus on something else to numb and avoid the reality that life can be tough, unfair, and downright difficult.

Meme, as my siblings and I lovingly called her, was not a distant grandmother who sent greeting cards in the mail and called only on birthdays. No, Meme was actively involved in my life and the lives of my siblings. She was our "get out of jail card" when breaking something in the house, as my siblings and I commonly did growing up. Any time we were in trouble for regular mischief of a child, one call to Meme, and the problem was solved. Our parents would extend us grace. In fact, one of our favorite things to do growing up was to have a "pajama ride" to Meme's house. What is a pajama ride, you ask? It is the brilliant idea my mother came up with to manage the bedtime routine of four small children—the three oldest, each two years apart, and the baby who joined the group five years after my arrival. This was the deal—a pajama ride could occur any day of the week (school nights included), unknown to us if we did the following. If my three siblings and I took the initiative and independently got ready for bed, showered, brushed our teeth, put our pajamas on by a certain time, then my mom would go into the hallway of our home with car keys in hand and shout "Pajama ride!" But here is the caveat—it was an all-or-none deal, even the baby. Now I realize this was to encourage the necessity to watch out for each other and help your siblings. When we heard those joyous words, "Pajama ride!" that was the indication that mom noticed the great responsibility we displayed and effort of working together and helping each other. This, however, is where I have to add that it was usually my older sister Tania helping me or my younger brother get ready for bed while big brother Nathan charged us on to move faster. "Pajama ride." At once, those unexpected two words would be followed by the sound of little feet scampering. My three siblings and I would come running from all different directions and jump in the backseat of the car while Mom drove to an undisclosed location. That location could be the local ice cream shop. We could go into the store in our pajamas and choose a table where all of us could gather around to enjoy our ice-cream cones. That location could be just a drive to downtown as my three siblings and I piled together in the back seat of the car and gaze out the window to see the lights and tall buildings and vicariously live the hustle and bustle of the adults we saw enjoying the night life. Or that location could be our very favorite, Meme's house. Meme would meet us at the door with a big smile and some sort of evening dessert in hand. A big hug followed, which became a rocking dance as she held each of us one by one tightly and close to her body. She expressed how proud she is of us and affirmed our action and decision in helping and encouraging each other to get ready for bed before our mom asked. Then we made our way to her living room. You know, the living room for the adults and guests, where prayer meetings would occur with the high-back furniture covered in plastic. Yes, that was the spot we as kids were allowed to sit and enjoy eating pastry cakes or cookies of "pajama ride" night. That is my Meme.

So at the start of my senior year of high school when my Meme was diagnosed with pancreatic cancer, my world began to shake and shift. The unknown was approaching my life head on. I did not share my emotional distress and mental uneasiness with anyone. Support was available in my home, at my local church, and at my alma mater Deerfield Beach High School. But instead, I chose to ignore the sadness and pain. I dug myself deeper in my studies. I trained harder on the track field to prepare for the state track completion, which I was for sure in because I was the only senior scholar athlete in my county who was competing at the state level since freshman year. In the middle of my senior year, the cancer spread in Meme's body. The chemotherapy treatment was not working. The decision was made to place Meme on hospice, since the medication would cause more damage to her healthy cells instead of eradicating the cancer cells. Then you could visibly see her short, round frame beginning to thin out. Her hands appeared weaker, and her bright eyes were slowly becoming dull. I was devastated, and still my response was to train harder, study harder, and push because I just did not want to think about or pay attention to the emotional turmoil within that began to produce physical pain in my abdomen. Meme's health continued to decline. My siblings and I lamented silently when we were alone and away from each other but became actors of great strength when we were all together. Before my senior year of high school was over, Meme breathed her last breath on earth and her first breath in heaven. I did not qualify for state track meet my senior year. My grade point average dropped in the last quarter of my senior year. Meme did not make it to my high school graduation. She was not present at Senior Awards Night to see the awards and scholarships I received to attend The University of Florida, and she was not there to see me all dressed up for my high school prom.

The complexities and connections of the human body are so amazing. The body is an interdependent system of physical health, spiritual health, and cognitive health that forgets nothing. When we do not address something in our lives, it does not just go away. It remains present, only unseen. It hides and manifests itself somewhere else in our body or in the future when dealing with a familiarity, it shows up again. For me, that unaddressed pain presented itself nine years later while in the rigors of medical school. A familiar emotion appeared afflicting my cognitive health. The provoking event leading to this distress was the sudden passing of my soon-to-be father-in-law from an automobile accident followed by the passing of my grandfather thirty days of later. This time, my will to be strong and keep pushing through to ignore the pain and sadness was not achievable. Believe me, I attempted. I said nothing to anybody, and it became increasingly difficult to concentrate on my studies and focus during lectures. As my grades began suffering, I was exposed. This time, I could not stay hidden. My hurt, pain, and natural expected heartache were exposed, and they had to be addressed appropriately.

I have witnessed this same interdependent system of our health play out when treating hospice patients. Individuals with emotional pain of unforgiveness or broken family relationships experience physical pain. Despite high doses of morphine or methadone around the clock, the patient continues to complain of pain. It is not until intentional, calculated, active steps are taken to seek out forgiveness or mend broken relationships that the physical pain begins to decrease. Likewise, there is growing literature regarding patients with devastating terminal diagnoses who choose optimism as the driving force of their Cognitive Health. Those patients report improved quality of life and decreased pain, and some outlive their prognosis.

As a Physician, I have seen clear evidence of cognitive health having a direct impact on a patient's physical health. When I unpack my personal experience of ignoring emotional distress, I realize its negative effect on my overall wellbeing. This leads me to the certainty that optimal health, or wholeness in our health, can only thrive when all three components of our health are routinely examined and addressed. Our physical health needs regular attention, just as our spiritual health should be routinely addressed, along with our cognitive health partaking in consistent assessment. Caring for only one of the three components that make up our health and overlooking the other two leaves us with unaddressed ailments that remain hidden all while producing signs and symptoms of illness. *The Healthy Whole Rx* was written to begin a conversation away from the default way health is defined and how it is addressed.

As for me, using the Healthy Whole Rx when it comes to my personal health has enabled me to live a life that is no longer fragmented. I am a wife, mom, physician, and friend. The cognitive demand on my mind requires me to set in place a protected time of mindfulness meditation in order to be available first for myself, then for my family, friends, and patients. The physical demand of raising three boys age eight, five, and two compels me to schedule routine visits with a physician and consistently make healthy lifestyle decisions that will enhance my productivity and energy. My spiritual need and dependence for a savior requires me to fill the God gap in my soul with the truth of His word. Yes, it takes strategic work that is possible and attainable. Are you overwhelmed with your health? Are you tired of living an unfulfilled life of more low points than highs? Have you had enough of the racing thoughts of anxiety that keep you up at night? If so, here is your solution. *The Healthy Whole Rx* is for you.

TAKE ACTION WITH HONEST REFLECTION

1. Is your default Nature Strength?

   Yes or No

2. What are you labeling as strength that is truly something you are subconsciously avoiding and not appropriately addressing?

____

____

____

____

____

____

The Purpose: First identify then address the natural hardships of life.

After addressing, develop the discipline to keep the disappointment in perspective.

To enhance your quality of life, practice being intentional and purposeful with yourself and those around you.

Notes

Notes

Notes

Notes

Notes

Notes

Notes

CHAPTER 2

Interdependent System of Health

What is physical health? Physical health is more than what you see reflected in the mirror. It includes our body's function and its ability in movement, flexibility, energy, and endurance. Our physical health oftentimes mistakenly carries the load—the heavy lifting in how we define and decide whether or not a person is healthy. Your physical health, of course, is influenced by genetics, family history, and even environment. However, there is more to the story. You need to know that there exists in your body and mine the reality that what we see or measure as physical health is also directly influenced and dependent on our spiritual and cognitive health.

What is spiritual health? Spiritual health is our need for and connection with our creator. Some will refer to spiritual health as the thing our soul needs in order to thrive and be happy and well. Unlike physical health, we cannot tangibly touch to feel spiritual health. In addition, we cannot see spiritual health, yet its role in the Healthy Whole Rx is foundational and essential. Your spiritual health depends on your intentional actions to remain connected with our creator, and only you can keep that connection to maintain your spiritual health. Spiritual health gives us purpose. It develops the narrative of why we are here on earth at this set time, in this set space, participating in these set things. Spiritual health places perspective and ease in our lives while lifting the self-imposed heavy burden to perform well and exceptionally in everything we do at all times in order to be accepted and validated by our peers and those around us. Wholeness in your spiritual health will transform the trajectory of your life.

What is cognitive health? Cognitive health is the health of our mind. Our mind is the most powerful organ in our body. The mind's ability to function drives and directs the moving physical parts of our body that creates and maintains life as we know it. Physical trauma to our brain (e.g. a stroke or other brain injury) can affect the function of our mind. But repetitive, small, *unaddressed* emotional trauma or disappointment can disrupt a healthy mind. Constant grinding with limited to no rest to achieve a set goal then immediate repetition of this cycle also inhibits a healthy mind. Cognitive health requires renewing your mind consistently and renewing your mind progressively. It requires the demand to control and take captive your thinking and what you are setting your mind on the most.

So what do you think about the most? Is it anxious thoughts of despair, misfortune, or danger? Are you thinking more about an unwanted health report? Do you spend more time thinking about the what ifs of your life? Does your mind carry a daily tasking burden that plays out the scenario of what if everything goes wrong, what if the worst occurs, what if...? My friend Lysa put it this way: "You will steer where you stare." Answer this question in this moment, right now. Be honest. In the last 24 hours, what was your mind staring at the most? If it was inundated with thoughts of past hurts and disappointments, broken relationships, and unwanted negative outcomes, then your mind is over-processing toxic, negative thoughts. But if in the last 24 hours you were recalling joyous occasions, expecting great outcomes, and looking forward to the future, then you will steer and create mindfulness that is positive and productive to your overall health. When we address our mind health, and actively practice mindfulness, we dismantle any of the toxic, negative thoughts that obstruct our overall wellbeing.

Three Points of the Triangle: The Healthy Rule of Three

Health is not simply the absence of disease. It is in fact an interdependent triad of physical health, spiritual health, and cognitive health. Think of a triangle. A triangle has three individual points, but those points are all connected. Pulling on one individual point of a triangle creates stress or change at the other two points, as is the case when we speak of our Health. To achieve wholeness in our health, we must first recognize our health as a triad—a triangle with physical health, spiritual health, and cognitive health as its points. And like with any triangle, pulling at the point of our cognitive health will create stress in our physical and spiritual health. Likewise, pulling at the point of our spiritual health will create stress in our physical and cognitive Health. And finally, pulling at the point of our physical health will create stress in our spiritual and cognitive health. The Healthy Whole Rx is this. You and I must bring and keep our physical health, spiritual health, and cognitive health in alignment. Alignment is the supportive positioning of the three components of our health.

When you think about your health, ask yourself these three questions.

Question 1) Is my physical health supporting my spiritual and cognitive health?

Question 2) Is my spiritual health developing my cognitive and physical health?

Question 3) Is my cognitive health helping my physical and spiritual health?

If you answered no to any one of those questions, then your health is fragmented. Fragmented health is like one area of health competing against the other two. And staying in constant competition in anything is tiring and downright draining. Fragmented health places sole emphasis on only one component of our health while disregarding the other two components. It hinders the communication and inter-reliant need and mission of our physical health, spiritual health, and cognitive health to connect and achieve wholeness. Daily we see the outcomes of fragmented health. What is the effect of fragmented health? Burnout. Let me explain. Remember that fragmented health competes with itself. In other words, your physical health competes with your spiritual health, which competes with your cognitive health, and they all compete with each other for attention and care. When you only pay attention to your physical health and neglect the needs of your cognitive health for mental breaks, your cognitive health reacts to this neglect by producing signs and symptoms of burnout. What are those signs or symptoms of burnout? Constant physical fatigue. I mean the type of fatigue where despite sleeping the entire night, you wake up tired. Another sign is clumsiness. Is your coordination off? Are you bumping into things more frequently throughout the day? Do you find that your mental capacity to recall things is not as sharp as it used to be? Does it now take you a lot more time to complete a written task at work? Are the home improvement projects you used to knock out in thirty to forty-five minutes tops now taking you hours to complete? If you answered yes to any of these questions, then this is the result of distress in your cognitive health, which is sending physical alarms to alert you of something that is wrong. Burnout stems from a lack of intentional measures to care for our mind and ignorance to the need of regular cognitive rest and elimination of toxic thought patterns frequently. But here is the good news. You are reading this book, and you hold in your hands the Healthy Whole Rx that will take your health from fragmented pieces to wholeness in health.

TAKE ACTION WITH HONEST REFLECTION

Respond to the following statements.

1. I want the freedom of having wholeness in my health and life.
    a. Yes
    b. No

2. I desire improved physical health and need to begin regular physical activity/exercise.
    a. Yes
    b. No

3. My spiritual health needs improvement.
    a. Yes
    b. No

4. My cognitive health is in need of regular intentional care.
    a. Yes
    b. No

5. The Healthy Whole Rx addressing physical health, spiritual health, and cognitive health is a strategy I am willing to try.
    a. Yes
    b. No

Notes

Notes

Notes

Notes

Notes

Notes

Notes

CHAPTER 3

Feed Your Physical Health

The first step in feeding your physical health is finding a physician. I am not talking about Dr. Google. You know Dr. Google. Be honest—you may be one of his most faithful clients. Every time you have a cough or cold, you grab your hand device, do a search on the symptoms, then treat yourself. While your steps to take action regarding your health are great, they are directed towards the wrong place. Listen, I would never go to my mechanic to get my hair done. Thus, you, too, cannot only seek out health care with an internet search engine. Again, you need a physician who is a good fit for you. A physician you feel comfortable asking questions. A physician to whom you can speak directly who understands you and you understand them. This is the essence of a healthy patient-physician relationship. I want to bring attention to this thought of establishing a relationship with a physician with whom you can speak to directly. For some people, a language barrier presents as a hindrance in communicating directly with their physician. Although translation lines are available in many outpatient offices, the common saying is true—some information gets "lost in translation." Keep this in mind when choosing a physician, but do not let this keep you from establishing care with a physician. Ask family or friends about their physician. They can provide insight on their experience or a recommendation. Do not just blindly choose your physician from the Yellow Pages (Does anyone still use the Yellow Pages?). The patient-physician relationship has to be a good fit.

Once you have decided on a physician, you now need at minimum an annual exam. This is often referred to an annual wellness check. This is the appointment where family history is discussed to identify any risk of disease or illness. This appointment also should focus on preventive measures. Preventive measures are in place to prevent illnesses or diseases. Many preventive measures go hand and hand with screenings or simple blood tests, many of which can be completed in your physician's office. Because medicine is not and should never be one size fits all, your discussion on preventive Health is based upon age, gender, ethnicity, and social factors, to name a few. This discussion begins to provide the framework and foundation in achieving wholeness in your health. Once all that information is gathered and screenings and blood test are completed, then results can be given at the follow-up visit. Do not skip the follow-up visit. This is where you get the blueprint of exactly what is occurring in your body.

Ignorance is *not* bliss. You need to know what is going on in your body. I love follow-up visits with my patients because they are educational. I love educating my patients. I get to provide my patients with a simple, concrete understanding of what's going on in their body and how it is affecting their wellbeing. It is where I get to map out with my patients health goals, roads to take, and valleys and ditches to avoid and alert them to possible hazards ahead. That's my analogy for a goals of care discussion. We go through practical everyday steps to achieving those goals and identification of unwholesome or unhealthy lifestyle behaviors and pinpoint my patients' specific risk of future disease based on the results of their blood work and family history to reach Wholeness in Health. Listen, friend. This is a conversation in which you have to actively take part, because it is your body and your health. Do not skip this follow-up visit. This is where you ask all the questions you have in order to better understand how to care for yourself.

Own your health. No excuses. In high school, I played basketball and ran track. On the track field, I learned life lessons thanks to a great coach, Sherman Morris. One of the lessons he drilled into my mind as a sixteen-year-old junior in high school was, "Excuses are tools of incompetence, and incompetence is never allowed." Education and your willingness to learn shatters incompetence. And so is true for your health. You can learn and implement healthy habits. You can own your health and know what is going on in your body. There exist unpreventable risk factors—things you cannot change—such as genetics or family history. But there also exist preventable risk factors that you can control. Preventable factors that you can change right now include lifestyle and exercise.

Exercise is a needed selfish act in which I encourage you to indulge. It is selfish because it is all about you. Your exercise schedule must remain self-seeking, egotistic, and self-regarding. I need you to be greedy in this case, setting a schedule to take care of yourself first, doctor's orders. Instead of being viewed as a need, exercise is often pushed aside as an extra thing we do if we have the time. Friend, the problem is that if you are waiting for that "if I have the time moment," it will never come. And sadly, you will gradually develop joint stiffness, which precedes aches and pains. Then ultimate sign of inactivity is the "Oh Jesus" when moving from a seated to standing position. The "Oh Boy" after only going up one flight of stairs. Or the "Whoy" when bending down to pick up a piece of paper. The "Oh Jesus," "Oh Boy" and "Whoy" are all preventable if you would just commit to being selfish with your exercise and prioritize yourself. You remember the story of the tortoise and the hare. It was the small, consistent steps that brought victory to tortoise. It was his commitment to small steps that produced a well-known victory during and after his life. A win that decades upon decades later we still know and talk about as a triumph that allowed for his name, Tortoise, to now appear in this book. Where will your name appear? Will it be your name and legacy that is passed down your family line? Will you be noted as the hero or heroine who changed the health trajectory of your family? They are watching in admiration, taking note of your commitment and action that is producing the results they see. Like Tortoise, bet on yourself and commit to small, consistent, selfish steps of exercise.

I know exercise sounds like work. Truly, it is, because like work, you have to be committed. But the base of exercise is movement. So instead of exercise, just do the physical activity you enjoy doing. If that is playing basketball, play basketball. If that is swimming, then swim. If that is dancing, then turn on that radio in your house three times a week and have a dance party with the family. Whatever it is, just get moving! Part of our physical health is the need to be up, active, and moving. When we stop moving, we start declining. Slowly, we lose body flexibility. When we become more sedentary, our fatigue level actually increases. So, this is what it comes down to. Cross out the excuses. ~~I am busy~~. ~~It looks like rain~~. ~~I have the kids with me.~~ ~~I am tired.~~ Just get out there and get moving!

TAKE ACTION: LET'S GET MOVING

This week, commit to doing the physical activity you enjoy doing.

Write down three physical activities you enjoy doing:

1. ______________________________

2. ______________________________

3. ______________________________

Now commit three days this week to doing thirty minutes of one of the listed activities above and have fun!

Day 1 ______________________________

Activity______________________________

Day 2 ______________________________

Activity______________________________

Day 3 ______________________________

Activity ______________________________

Notes

Notes

Notes

Notes

Notes

Notes

Notes

CHAPTER 4

Feed Your Spiritual Health

Connect to Your Creator to Know Your Identity

Here is the truth, and into it He blew the breath of life, and man became a living soul. You were created by God. There is a God hole inside of you and me that can only be filled by God. The creation needs to connect with its Creator. These are not just words that sound good. We see it in nature all the time. A baby lion cub upon birth immediately looks to make its his way to his mother to nurse. A newborn baby is placed on the belly of his mother and instinctively begins movement towards the breast of his mother. The creation has a need to be connected to the creator. The truth tells us that we were created in the image of God. Our souls fight everything we see and hear as we live out life in this fallen world. Our soul attempts to pull out the truth to heal the deep wounds, scars, and lies of inadequacy, inability, and defeat that can come in this life. The lies that stand to blind confuse and destroy your soul. And it is for this very reason that you must feed your spiritual health with the truth. Feed your spiritual health with the truth that you are created in the image of God, that in you, there is nothing missing, nothing lacking. Feed your spiritual health with the truth that you are strategically and wonderfully made for this moment, for your space, for a time such as this. It is only with the daily doses of the truth that we can be healthy and whole. Connecting to our creator gives God access to our souls to provides us with our identity and reminds us of who we really are. And who are you? You are created for a purpose, chosen, loved by God, with great ability to be healthy and whole. God has a good plan for you despite what has happened, despite what you have participated in, despite what those closest to you say. He says, "You are mine, and I love you." He wants to feed your spiritual health. Your stance and position is to just let Him do it. Grant Him access to you as He feeds you Biblical truths that override and supersede the facts.

My friend Lysa says it is vital to our everyday life that we "listen to the whispers of God before we hear the shouts of the world." That we tune into His promise of protection, His instruction for our day to feed our spiritual health. Those quiet moments in the morning when you first wake up and lying still in bed is the opportune time for prayer and devotion. Prayer is a personal conversation, spoken or unspoken, between you and God. Now truly, I have never heard the audible voice of God, but what I have experienced is a sense of direction; a deep-rooted feeling of peace regarding a matter that was troubling my soul. "Do not be anxious about anything, but in every situation, by prayer and petition, with thanksgiving, present your requests to God. And the peace of God, which transcends all understanding, will guard your hearts and your minds in Christ Jesus" (Philippians 4: 6-7, NIV). The amount and depth of brokenness I see in the hearts of man as a doctor made me quickly realize medication alone was not enough. I began to pull and give my patients the prescription that was given to me growing up as a daughter of a Baptist reverend and a mother who constantly pointed us to her need and ours for Jesus Christ. Whether it was hosting prayer meetings in our home, family devotion around our parents' bed, or transparent discussions of their peace and hope in the midst of chaos, what I now understand was occurring was consistent food and attention to our spiritual health. Prayer and devotion are a committed consecrated time where you communicate with God and He with you. This, too, is a needed selfish act that should be seen as scared, uncompromising "me time" to feed your soul and ultimately address your spiritual health.

It is not good for man to be alone. We were all created to be in community and relationship with others. We see this happen in medicine—the onset of depression that walks hand and hand with individuals who live lives that are isolated from others. No, it is not good for man to be alone. We all need a community, a tribe, a family on which we can lean. A group of people that will support us, individuals who will cry with us when life brings disappointments and rejoice with us when life brings joy and victory. There is a story I love in the Bible about a group of friends who literally (not figuratively) carried their sick friend to Jesus. The crowd was so great that they could not get in. I imagine them looking for a back door or side door and still not finding a way to get inside. In this time, they looked at the face of the friend that they carried all day with hope that their sick friend would be made healthy and whole. That paralyzed man who was carried by his friends to Jesus left the presence of Jesus walking out healthy and whole. But how did he finally get through the crowd? What made the difference? Those friends viewed their friend's infirmity as their own. And when they could not get through the front door the traditional route, they scaled the wall, put a hole in the roof, and lowered him to the feet of Jesus. Those are the kind of friends you need, the type of support you need, and the specific prayer you should pray, because it is not good for man to be alone.

I am reminded of three of my closest friends Tane, Nikcy, and Nickline. They are my sister friends. We have known each other since middle school. Life has taken us to highs of establishing businesses and wedding receptions, but this same life has taken us to the miscarriage of twin babies, the hospital rooms for chronic illnesses, and each other's living rooms where together we go to God in prayer and petition with thanksgiving for healing our children or parents who are ill. It is not good for man to be alone. There can be times in this life where you will not have the strength to carry yourself, but before that happens, you need a support network. Just as I have with my sister friends and just as this man had in this story, you, too, need a backing that will drive you towards spiritual health.

Know the truth, and the truth will set you free. There is a greater truth that we must affirm in our hearts, soul, and mind. It is the biblical truths—affirmations of who God said we are, what He promises he will do, and His intention for us to live life fearlessly. These affirmations can be found in the GPS guide for your life and mine that we call the Bible. It is amazing how difficult situations will cause you to search for and develop a skill that you never knew you had or could do. As you know from this chapter, I grew up across the hall from the pastor, and if there was one thing we had in abundance in our house it was Bibles. To this day, you can go to my parents' home and find multiple versions of the Bible in English, French, Haitian Creole, and Hebrew. And we would sing that well-known children's song, "Read your Bible prayer every day, and you'll grow, grow, grow." Growing up, the Bible was the last thing I desired to read. But when my firstborn encountered a situation that disrupted his confidence and countenance, how quickly I grabbed a Bible. During that time, my son began to complain of back aches, stomach aches, or some sort of ailment when getting ready for school. That was followed by the statement, "Mommy, I can't go to school today." Well, after asking more questions and talking to him, his teacher, and the principal, we realized that as a first grader at the tender age of six years old, he was being bullied. Okay. This is where I just have to interrupt my typing and your reading and say that no six-year-old should be inventing ways to stay home from school because he is fearful of a bully. Now back to our discussion. We advocated on his behalf, made changes, spoke with him, and reminded him the he was safe. Yet months later, his confidence and countenance were still fragmented and shaky. Our fearless, outspoken, outgoing, talkative extrovert was becoming silent, hidden, and full of fear. At that point I did for him what my parents did for me daily. I spoke Biblical affirmations to him right before he walked into the doors of the school. It did not take me long to grab a few of those Bibles around my house, place them on the kitchen table, and write on notecards and sticky notes what God affirms to be True for Baylen's life and my shaking heart. I now say these affirmations to all of my boys, and they say them to each other (the two-year-old makes an attempt). So if you ever see me dropping off my clan of three at the front gates of their school, this is what you will hear: "Baylen, you are a man of integrity and character. You will bless the Lord at all times, and God's Praise will forever be on your lips. The enemy is a defeated foe in your life. You wear the full armor of God. You have the mind of Christ. You have the wisdom of God, and you operate in it. Bay, you are the head and not the tail, above and not beneath, the lender and never the borrower. You are a leader among men, and you lead your people in love and Godly works. And Bay, God has an amazing plan for your life. And now you tell me about the plan of the Lord." Baylen answers, "The plans of the Lord stand firm forever" (Psalms 33:11, NIV). That's who you are, Baylen, and do not ever forget it." After a month of this daily reminder, my baby got his confidence back. It is time for you to discover the Biblical affirmations that will feed your spiritual health to shatter toxic negative doubts and any patterns of self-destruction. The nourishment for our heart and the strength for our soul starts when we affirm who we are.

Feeding our spiritual health can also occur in the form of what we are listening to and what we are watching. Okay, if you are this far in the book, I feel safe to have a moment of confessions with Dr. Sabine Elisee. Every now and then, I enjoy pointless television. Especially after having a critical day where I had to start CPR on a patient to save their life, surely I earned a moment of pointless television. But my hubby hates it for very clear reasons. He is convinced that many pointless reality shows kill brain cells the longer you sit and watch them. And the discussion at that moment when pointless television is on in the home of Team Elisee is, "Babe, you know the longer you watch this, the more your intelligence will decrease." I say this because there is some truth in his thoughts. Visual and audible stimuli influence our wellbeing. It has happened to you before, I am sure. You had a day that was more difficult than usual, you are feeling a little down, then as you are sitting in the car on your drive home, a song you love comes on the radio, and suddenly you start rocking your head to the beat and singing. What you are hearing is feeding your soul with encouragement that evoked a smile, head bop, and songs to come forth and pass through your lips. On those drives in the car, and especially as you start your day, make intentional decisions to feed your spiritual health through what you are hearing. Maybe you are in a season of your life where the demands of aging parents, young children, or a business to operate can limit a formal quiet sit-down at the office table to feed your spiritual health. Your Rx, friend, is to integrate. As you are getting ready for work, preparing meals, or on your drive, choose to listen to encouraging affirmations, transformational sermons, praise, or worship music that will allow access for God's peace and direction to steer your day. This is not impossible. You can integrate. While in medical school and residency, I learned how to integrate and identify what was most important in that season of life. We can only keep up with but so many things at a time. Even the virtuous woman that we read about in Proverbs 31 surely did not do all those things at one time. Instead, it was at different stages, different seasons in her life. I assure you of this because if she had done it all at once, that section of the Bible would be titled *The Burnt-Out Woman,* not *The Virtuous Woman*. In residency, I had 24-hour call shifts. Yes, that's right—a 2 and a 4 placed next to each other. For 24 hours, you cannot leave the hospital. In addition, I was recently married with a one-year-old driving 112 miles round trip five days a week, sometimes six, to the hospital where I was completing my residency training. During that time, I began to feel the symptoms of burnout seeking to pitch a tent in my life. One of those days, a patient noticed the fatigue on my face and reminded me to feed my spiritual health. As I began to tell her the reality of my busy schedule, she agreed that this season of my life had many responsibilities, but I could not neglect my spiritual health. Her recommendation was that on those long drives to play teaching and affirming messages that would strengthen my soul. Over the next three years of residency, I listened to some of my favorite speakers so much that it felt like they became friends who were in the car with me on my daily long drives. That small intentional adjustment made a difference in bringing fullness to my spiritual health. If you are looking for some driving friends, you can borrow mine—Karen Loritts, Barbara Rainey, Pricilla Shirer, and Lysa TerKeurst (yes, that would be my friend Lysa I mentioned earlier). Doctor's orders—do not just stop there in feeding your spiritual health. Add visuals. During that same time, the interior of my car became what looked like a war zone for sticky notes. I wrote reminders as they came. Sticky notes of encouraging verses, notecards of affirming truths, and promises of God were posted everywhere in my car.

TAKE ACTION: TRUTH > FACTS

Write five truths that you will repeat to yourself each day this week.

I am ____________________________________

I am ____________________________________

I am

I am

I am

Notes

Notes

Notes

Notes

Notes

Notes

Notes

CHAPTER 5

Feed Your Cognitive Health

Feeding your cognitive health requires needed selfish acts of meditation. Meditation differs from prayer and devotion in that mediation is a focused, engaged time of reflection. Mindfulness meditation can happen at any moment in your day. In the Healthy Whole Rx, it is necessary to be mindful of your emotions. Our emotions make up who we are. They tell the story of our lives, and we as individuals must decide what story our mind is telling us. Repetitive stories of hurt, pain, disappointment, fear, anxiety, and injustice are toxic to our mind. Those experiences have to be identified and dumped to support cognitive health. Daily mindfulness meditation is the best way to be aware and keep those toxic storehouses out of our mind. Early morning meditation to begin your day has helped people organize thoughts to prepare and frame up their day in their mind. Evening meditation can be beneficial to detox your mind of upsetting events of the day, recognize achievements, and more importantly, identify the present emotional state of your cognitive health. Our cognitive health is a driving force of our lives. Daily reflection is necessary. Is your cognitive health in a state of fatigue? Then rest your mind. Is your cognitive health in a state of sadness? Then identify what is the disappointment that occurred recently or even years ago that is causing this sadness. Interestingly, the alarm that our cognitive health needs attention does not sound until the toxicity in our mind begins to spill over—when sadness becomes depression and depression becomes a violent act of self-inflicted trauma, or worse, loss of life. The Healthy Whole Rx at the onset of a health assessment takes into account mind health and emotions to prevent devastating health outcomes. We never think of the role of cognitive health until it presents itself through symptoms of neglect. The person who always has makeup on suddenly is not wearing any lipstick. The man who always has a clean shave and an exact tapeline begins to have an "I do not care" attitude about his appearance.

These signs are more obvious. The signs that go unseen and unnoticed and remain under the radar are in the individuals who are excellent performers. To the men and women who are surrounded by many yet suffer silently and alone by hiding their tears and anxiety because they are top-notch performers, this section of this book is for you. I worry about you. The individuals I meet who are highly successful in their careers tend to need more focused discussion surrounding their cognitive health. Their anxiety and fear are because of the question of whether they will truly be able to keep up with their current level of success. They worry about having reached a plateau in their career and are now left with toxic, overwhelming thoughts that cycle in their mind night after night. Cognitive health begins with the engagement of mindfulness meditation to prevent the toxic thoughts that pollute our minds.

You must bring rest to your mind. Regular doses of brain rest is necessary. You and only you are the keeper of your brain. If you do not bring rest to your brain, it will continue to race and run. Imagine track and field runners who line up to start the open quarter race (one lap around the track). Runners take their marks, get set, and the gun goes off. The race begins, and quickly, the runners are rounding the last turn, approaching the finish line. Only they are not slowing down. They keep running. Lap after lap, they just keep running. Never stopping, they continue at the same pace going around and around and around. What will happen? Eventually, they will tire out. Their muscles will not be able to keep up with that pace. Such is the same for our minds. We were not made with the capacity to keep going like the energizer bunny in the commercials of the 80s. Think about it. God Himself rested on the seventh day. If He rested, then surely you and I must learn to bring rest to our minds. An unrested mind creates illness in our cognitive health.

Many people have learned how to multitask, but no one—absolutely no one—can multi-focus. There are certain events, moments, and assignments in your life that require your undivided attention. As a doctor, it would be detrimental to my patient if I dare multi-focus while writing a prescription. When you are driving in your car, please do not attempt to multi-focus on driving and reading news feeds. Cognitive health requires us to be fully present in the moment we are in, to minimize multiple stimuli. Like our cell phones and computers, which go slower when many windows are open, such is the case with our minds. While our mind is the strongest organ in our body, it cannot function at its peak capacity when we constantly place a demand on it to multi-focus.

Being fully present in the moment is especially important when spending time with loved ones, family members, or friends. One of the biggest regrets people share with me is not spending enough uninterrupted quality time with loved ones. Not only do our minds need this constructive nourishment, those moments train our minds to focus on one subject and emotion at a time. The five love languages describe how we as human beings receive and give love. Each of the five languages has a descriptive action that list how it is expressed or spoken. Quality time is one of the five love languages. The description of quality time is foundational and specific in the fact that this time cannot be split shared or in competition with anything else. If that occurs, then it is not the essence of quality time. The love language of our cognitive health is quality time.

In this age of hustle and bustle, there are many good and important things to do, but they may not be the best thing for you at the moment. There are many things that vie for our attention, including personal and familial responsibilities, work demands, social demands, community demands, and philanthropic causes. While they are all great, they cannot be addressed without mother wisdom being part of the conversation. Wisdom is the ability to make a decision of the day's activities with good judgment. Our cognitive health endures extensive strain from the endless demands we place on it due to a lack of wisdom. Doctor's orders—place a limit on that daily to-do list and the self-imposed desire to say yes to every request. The sooner you learn this and practice this cognitive health prescription, the sooner you will have better, lasting results of a healthy mind in the long term. "My mouth will speak words of wisdom. The meditation of my heart will give you understanding" (Psalms 49:3, NIV).

The mind thrives with factual information and understanding. Misleading, isolated, and absolute thinking will contaminate our minds. My five-year-old is in a phase where he speaks in absolutes when he gets upset with us. The conversation will sound like this: "Mommy, I want an Oreo for dinner." "No, Blakie, you have to eat real food for dinner." And as soon as he hears that two-letter word "No," he begins to rant and rave. Then comes the repeated song of "You never give me Oreo cookies. You never give me Oreo cookies." Well, you and I both know that just is not true. Blake would not know that he loves Oreo cookies if I never gave him Oreo cookies. But in that moment, he is convinced in his mind of this isolated absolute statement that is simply a lie. Even as adults, we have to be careful of those moments that creep into our minds. Those statements of "This never works out for me," "I am always losing my things," "I never get a good deal," and "They always leave me out and forget to call me to for dinner" are absolute negative statements that feed toxicity to our brain and create debility in our mind and cognitive health. At all costs, avoid these and similar isolated absolute toxic statements.

When, not if, disappointment, discouragement, anxiety, fear, or sadness comes in, your mind recognizes it. You must quickly recognize and identify those feelings to address them correctly. As I write this section of this chapter, it is as if I can hear my mom saying, "Sabi, you just can't bury your head in the sand and ignore the stressors that are going on in your life. You have to address them." And I submit to you this same pearl. Give attention to the stressors that have or are occurring in your life. One of the main reasons people suffer with insomnia is unaddressed stressors that create unhealthy underlying emotions that are at constant play in their subconscious. Our time for restorative rest that should occur when we sleep is hindered secondary to unaddressed and sometimes unidentified stressors that have attached to the circuits of our mind. When we sweep emotional distress under the rug, it only shows up somewhere else in our lives, remaining hidden, untreated, and masked, yet producing disjointed broken health.

Remember Blakie? When Blakie gets in the rant of "You never give me Oreo cookies," the only way to get him out of it is to redirect and capture his attention on that which is true.

We have discussed what is toxic to our brain, but we have to spend time outlining what is nourishing and healthy to our brain. We have to train our brains to focus on positive, enhancing thoughts. That which is constructive builds confidence, is helpful, and is encouraging. I call it my Practical Practice Plan based on this truth in Philippians 4:8 (NIV): "Finally, brothers and sisters, whatever is true, whatever is noble, whatever is right, whatever is pure, whatever is lovely, whatever is admirable—if anything is excellent or praiseworthy—think about such things." Our minds drive us in one of two directions—towards wholeness in our health or away from wholeness in our health. Dr. Elisee's signature Practical Practice Plan trains our mind to focus on and rehearse positive thoughts when feelings of fear or anxiety over take our minds. The word PLAN in the Practical Practice Plan is an acronym. It is a reminder to practice focusing our minds on thoughts that are Praiseworthy or Pure, Lovely, Admirable, and Noteworthy or Noble. Refocusing our thoughts reminds our brain that life comes with highs and lows. Spending more time cycling thoughts through our mind that are good develops our cognitive health.

The second half of the Practical Practice Plan is to practice gratitude. At the end each day, write down what went well in the last twenty-four hours. It can be as simple as "The coffee barista at my local coffee shop made my coffee just right" or "I received a call from my adult child to whom I have not spoken in weeks." It takes regime to train our minds in practicing gratitude. The more we practice gratitude, the easier it becomes. When gratitude becomes easy and automatic, it is at that point that a shift occurred in our mind. The Practical Practice Plan transforms our minds to a new pattern—a default nature that sees a new perspective and brings wholeness to our cognitive health.

TAKE ACTION: MINDFULNESS MEDITATION

Stop, Pause, Reflect

Sit outside in nature with a notebook or just this book.

First, give your mind the ability to identify three areas in your life that are troubling. Be specific and write them down. Writing them down allows your mind to take action and dump those thoughts.

1. ______________________________

____

____

____

____

2. ______________________________

____

____

____

____

3. ______________________________

____

____

____

____

Now that you have written them, if you have a solution, write it in the space below. If not, simply write "not yet." Also note that a solution can be a decision to see how this plays out or continue to pray and choose optimism.

1. ______________________________

____

____

2. ______________________________

____

____

3. ____

____

____

Finally, gratitude practice.

Identify and write five things for which you are grateful at this very moment.

1. ____

____

____

____

____

2. ____

____

____

____

____

3. ____

____

____

____

____

4. ____

____

____

____

____

5. ____

____

____

____

____

For the next 10-15 minutes, hyper focus and take in every sound you hear as you sit in nature.

Notes

Notes

Notes

Notes

Notes

Notes

Notes

CHAPTER 6

Discipline and Consistency

Indiscipline is the enemy of progress. Growing up in South Florida, on Saturday mornings, our house was filled with the sounds of the record player playing a popular Haitian band of the 70s called *Frere Parent*. My dad loves this band and still takes the time to explain the significance of their music that speaks of social injustice, the need for education, and expectation of each individual listening to build your community and strengthen your country and your fellow man. One of their songs has the chorus, "Indisipline lenmi pwogre, fok ou mete lode nan lavi ou." Translation: "Indiscipline is the enemy of progress, you must place order in your life." The statement is profound, and it has to settle within before it can expressed outwardly in thought and action. Good health takes consistent discipline. No quick shake or injection will achieve the lasting results for your health that you are seeking. Only self discipline to take consistent small steps towards your health can establish lasting results. The disconnect is that many people want wholeness in their health but live and establish their lives in the suburbs of indiscipline.

How do you become disciplined in your lifestyle? You think of and establish the healthy choices you will make regarding your physical, spiritual, and cognitive health today. Then you repeat this the next day, then the next, until finally, it becomes second nature. Here is an example of what that may look like. Wake up and address your spiritual health by reading one Biblical truth and taking a moment to think about it. Then make a decision to address your physical health. Perhaps it is a day that your schedule is full. Well, today, choose to park further away from any building you are going to enter. Make a decision to eat smaller, more frequent meals throughout the day and drink more water. Finally, address your cognitive health at the end of the day. Take a quiet moment for mindfulness meditation, then write out three things that occurred in the last twenty-four hours for which you are grateful.

Discipline carries wholeness to your health. Proverbs 5:23 (NIV) reminds us, "For lack of discipline they will die, led astray by their own great folly." Do not despise discipline, friend. If the most recent NFL Championship team despised disciple, they would have never achieved the victory on Super Bowl Sunday. If you despise discipline, you will never achieve wholeness in your health. The sacrifice it takes to bring discipline to your body, your spirit, and your mind will enhance your physical health, spiritual health, and cognitive health. We can no longer be slaves to our bodies. We cannot be held hostage by the fluctuating emotions of our soul. We cannot allow toxic thoughts patterns to erect contaminated communities in our minds. The Healthy Whole Rx teaches to eliminate all tools of incompetence—what we lightly label as being busy. The Healthy Whole Rx rests on our need for connection to our creator. The Health Whole Rx teaches to take captive toxic thoughts and dump them out of our brain to create a sound mind. The Healthy Whole Rx brings our physical health, spiritual health, and cognitive health in alignment to yield health and wholeness.

TAKE ACTION

Write three ways you will give attention to your physical health today, followed by three ways you will give attention to your spiritual health today, and finally, three ways you will give attention to your cognitive health today.

Physical Health

1. ____

____

____

____

2. ____

____

____

____

3. ____

____

____

____

Spiritual Health

1. ____

____

____

____

2. ____

____

____

____

3. ____

____

____

____

Cognitive Health

1. ____

____

____

____

2. ____

____

____

____

3. ____

____

____

____

Notes

Notes

Notes

Notes

Notes

Notes

Notes

Afterword

To the patients I have met at office visits, in fellowship halls of churches, and at health fairs. To the men and women of the beautiful country of Haiti who allowed me to care for their health needs at a Medical Missions trip. To the patients I meet in the hospital and those whose homes I go into. Thank you for allowing me to serve as your physician. I see you attempting to figure out and get better control of your health. I have listened to your stories of frustration and of not knowing what else to do. I have heard your passionate prayers for healing and direction. May the Healthy Whole Rx bring insight, direction, and answers to your prayers.

About the Author

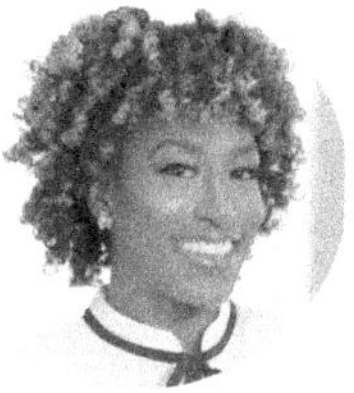

Dr. Sabine Elisee is a board-certified family medicine physician and certified health education specialist who earned her undergraduate degree in health science education from the University of Florida and her master's in public health and doctor of osteopathic medicine from Dr. Kiran C. Patel College of Osteopathic Medicine. Her biggest passions are providing people with tools to make informed choices about their health and helping them connect the fragmented pieces of their lives to enjoy wholeness. She enjoys playing basketball, going to the theatre, sitting on the beach, spending time with family and friends, and praying. She also enjoys volunteering at her church and community health fairs and mentoring pre-med college students.

Dr. Elisee is married to her husband, Vicly, and has three sons—Baylen, Blake, and Braxton. She lives in South Florida.

Learn more at www.DrSabineElisee.com